Title:

Fixing Myself

By Daniel Akol.

QUOTE:

"If you know how to read and don't read, then you are not different from the person who doesn't know how to read"

Table of Contents:

Introduction

Chapter 1: What Are Allergies?

Chapter 2: Common Allergens

Chapter 3: Signs and Symptoms of Allergies

Chapter 4: Diagnosing Allergies

Chapter 5: Allergy Testing Methods

Chapter 6: Treatment Options for Allergies

Chapter 7: Allergy Prevention and Management

Chapter 8: Where do allergies most likely show up?

Chapter 9: fasting for cell recycling.

Chapter 10: training to refer the damage tissues

Chapter 11: drinking water (staying hydrated)

chapter 12: protecting the skins

Conclusion.

What to expect: Diagnosing Common Allergies: Understanding the Causes and Finding Relief

Stay hydrated all the times*

Introduction:

Allergies affect millions of people worldwide, causing discomfort and interfering with daily life. From seasonal allergies to food sensitivities, understanding the causes and finding effective relief is essential for those who suffer from allergic reactions. "Diagnosing Common Allergies: Understanding the Causes and Finding Relief" explores the intricate world of allergies, providing comprehensive information on how to identify, diagnose, and manage common allergies. This book aims to empower individuals by equipping them with the knowledge to take control of their allergies and live a healthier, more comfortable life.

WINDOW ONE:

This book is written by Daniel Akol Kuan to help release the world from prison that the finds themselves in when they were born by their parents that have been born in the same cycle of imprisonment, so to start with this chapter I have to explain my jail experience and how I found the key to unlock the prison, I'm a young individual who have been born to poor family in south Sudan who have little or no resource or any educational background in any field, therefore it gives them many reasons to accept whatever is been told them by their parent and people around them, with less hesitation and fear of missing out, and the follow the rat race without questioning anything.

About me:

I was born in poor conditions in the month of march with little or no confirmed known allergies but as I began to grow the unexplainable changes began to manifest along the way and I began to question myself, why do I have this kind of problem that I can't even verify? I left with my mind riddling on what should be the cause and I know deep down in my heart that it's not what my parents or doctor claim to be.

Most of the time every second and third party {parents and doctors} might be guessing without accurate conclusion, therefore you must be the one to slowly but surely find when the issue arises and find the solution which will not only help you but others as well and if you are a parent you can apply this technique to deliver your young toddlers and animals who doesn't have the brain capacity to apply the technique on their own.

For me it was dairy products, milk and boil eggs as a whole that were triggering my reactions but when I found out I cut them off for good and since then I never been the same, I'm feeling energetic and amazing than never before I also watch out for potential triggers.

First of all whenever the problem arises whether it be headache, sore throat, acne, stomach issue, anxiety, and nerve issues.

The first thing you can ask is why does this start in the first place? And there are many factors that will be the root cause, what you need to do is to rewind back to whatever the last thing you have done and the last place you have been.

Short story:

 that I witness was: a young child was being taken care of by a sister who is older than him and one day they were outside the house 2 km away from home and as they were playing in the old garden of groundnut, the caretaker had left his little brother and went to play with her peers for the moment and as she was there she heard his brother screaming and crying, so she ran to see what was going on, as she arrived in the scene, she see her brother not breathing normally and his mouth was wide open with his hand on his neck trying to say that there was something on his throat but because he was 17 months old he couldn't communicate but point at his neck, people have become frustrated and confused on what happened to him, I was one of them and a lot of scenarios where made but no conclusion or solution to be reached and so the clock is ticking for the innocent child, the whole town was there witnessing the scene, but my question was, where was you and the child when this happened I ask the caretaker and she said, on the old garden

Me: Were you separated from him at any time?

Her: yes but not much

And because I was working on the pharmacy and knew more about the environment situation, I began to connect the dots and my scenario was that, this child was probably playing and he saw anything on the ground and picked up and as you might guess all living things specifically youngsters only know eating, he might have put something on his mouth and swallowed it causing him to suffocate, so I performed some exercises on him, I let him sips some milk because they like milk and he couldn't breathe or accept milk, I had to just pour them into his mouth and close his mouth for a little and turn him upside down, and miraculously the small cactus plant fall out from his throat, letting him breathe instantly and began to search for his mother breast, it was a big relief from the whole small town ended, therefore you always needed to approach the issue from the starting point

" No matter how bad you try, you can't help the person who doesn't want to help themselves, every good idea you make to them is a trigger to their beliefs system " Daniel Akol.

Don't be afraid to ask questions

"Asking question is not doubting, by not asking questions you will begin to doubt whether you've been lie to or you are going in right directions" therefore asking question to know whether you're working in correct way or not will not only save you but will save whoever was leading you if you turn out to be right, isn't that worth questioning everything?

Here are the question you might ask:

Who is influencing me?

Why am I eating this type of food and who told me to do so?

If I can live without this { sugar, cigarette, alcohol, vape, energy drink, etc} why would I need them now?

When this pain started, what was the last thing I did?

Why am I doing what I'm doing now is it because of my parents or my friends and if so can i decide on my own?

How was my childhood?

Are there any genetic or chronic illnesses with my parents if you witness both of your parents alive and how to minimise them from influencing you? If you didn't witness your parents how to assess the situation and come up with a solution?

Does someone else{doctor, foreteller, advisors, etc} know more about my body than I do, if not can I be a sole decision maker and put them in a third party position?

What if I can find my own way of living life?

Why am I applying this make-up, is it because everyone is wearing them or do I have my personal issues and if I have my personal issues, what are they and how can I address them in a natural way?

And

You can add more questions in this blank space and find the answers to them and be your own friend before anyone.

Assess before medication:

Whenever something arises whether be acne or any discomfort in body, our intuition quickly says there's something wrong with our bodies and doctors are ready to give you medicine

In this opening chapter, we will delve into the fascinating world of allergies, exploring what they are and how they affect the body. Allergies are the result of an overactive immune system's response to typically harmless substances, known as allergens. These substances can vary widely, ranging from pollen and pet dander to certain foods and medications.

Understanding the immune system's role in allergies is crucial to grasp the underlying mechanisms at play. When an allergen enters the body, it triggers an immune response, leading to the release of histamines and other chemicals that cause the characteristic allergic reactions. These reactions can manifest in various ways, such as pimples, sneezing, itching, hives, or even life-threatening anaphylaxis.

Allergies can develop at any age, and individuals may develop new sensitivities over time. While some allergies are hereditary, others may be acquired through repeated exposure or environmental factors. It is important to note that allergies are not curable, but with proper management and treatment, symptoms can be alleviated to provide relief.

Window Two:

Chapter 1: what are allergies?

Allergies occur when the immune system mistakenly identifies a usually harmless substance as a threat and reacts by producing antibodies called Immunoglobulin E (Ige). These antibodies cause certain cells to release chemicals, such as histamine, which lead to allergy symptoms.

This book will sets the foundation for understanding allergies, laying the groundwork for the subsequent exploration of common allergens, signs and symptoms, diagnostic techniques, and treatment options. By comprehending the basics of allergies, readers will be better equipped to navigate the journey towards diagnosis and relief.

In the next chapter, we will explore the most common allergens that individuals encounter in their daily lives. From airborne allergens like pollen and dust mites to food allergens such as peanuts and shellfish, understanding the sources of allergens is essential in identifying potential triggers. We will delve into the prevalence of each allergen, their potential effects on the body, and ways to minimise exposure.

Stay tuned for Chapter 2: Common Allergens, where we dive deeper into the world of allergens and their impact on allergic individuals.

Chapter 2: Common Allergens

In this chapter, we will explore the wide array of common allergens that individuals encounter in their daily lives. By understanding these allergens, we can gain insights into their prevalence, effects on the body, and methods to minimise exposure.

1. Pollen:

Pollen is one of the most common allergens, especially during certain seasons. It is produced by plants for reproduction and is carried by the wind or insects. When individuals with pollen allergies come into contact with pollen, it triggers an allergic reaction, leading to symptoms such as sneezing, itchy eyes, and a runny nose. Common sources of pollen allergies include trees, grasses, and weeds.

2. Dust Mites:

Dust mites are microscopic creatures that thrive in warm and humid environments. They are commonly found in bedding, upholstered furniture, and carpets. Allergic reactions to dust mites can include sneezing, coughing, wheezing, and itchy skin. Reducing exposure to dust mites through regular cleaning, using allergen-proof bedding, and maintaining low humidity levels can help alleviate symptoms.

3. Pet Dander:

Pet dander consists of tiny flakes of skin, saliva, and urine from animals such as cats, dogs, and rodents. Allergies to pet dander can cause symptoms ranging from sneezing and coughing to skin rashes and difficulty breathing. It is important for individuals with pet allergies to limit exposure by keeping pets out of certain areas of the home, regularly cleaning and vacuuming, and considering allergy-friendly pets or hypoallergenic breeds.

4. Mould:

Mould is a type of fungus that thrives in damp and humid environments. It can be found both indoors and outdoors, particularly in areas with moisture problems such as bathrooms, basements, and kitchens. Mould allergies can lead to symptoms such as sneezing, congestion, and respiratory issues. Preventing mould growth through proper ventilation, reducing moisture, and promptly addressing water leaks is crucial in managing mould allergies.

5. Food Allergens:

Food allergies are common, and certain foods can trigger allergic reactions in susceptible individuals. Some common food allergens include peanuts, tree nuts, shellfish, dairy products, eggs, wheat, and soy. Food allergies can cause symptoms ranging from mild itching and hives to severe reactions like anaphylaxis. Identifying and avoiding trigger foods is essential, and individuals with food allergies should always read food labels carefully and communicate their allergies to restaurants and food establishments.

6. Insect Stings:

Insect stings from bees, wasps, hornets, and fire ants can cause allergic reactions. For individuals with insect sting allergies, a single sting can result in a severe allergic reaction, including swelling, difficulty breathing, and in rare cases, anaphylaxis. It is important for those with insect sting allergies to be aware of their triggers, carry emergency medication (such as epinephrine), and seek immediate medical attention if stung.

Understanding these common allergens is a crucial step in identifying potential triggers and managing allergies effectively. In Chapter 3, we will explore the signs and symptoms of allergies, providing a comprehensive understanding of how allergies manifest in the body. Stay tuned for an in-depth exploration of the diverse range of allergic reactions and their impact on individuals' well-being.

7.Nuts allergies that most people don't know:

There are many different types of nuts, each with its own unique characteristics and flavours. Here are some common types of nuts:

1. Almonds: Almonds are a popular nut known for their mild, slightly sweet taste. They are often eaten raw, roasted, or used in various forms such as almond butter or almond milk.

2. Walnuts: Walnuts have a rich, slightly bitter taste and are often used in baking or as a topping for salads or oatmeal. They are a good source of omega-3 fatty acids.

3. Cashews: Cashews have a buttery, creamy flavour and are often eaten roasted or used in cooking, particularly in Asian cuisine. They can also be processed into cashew butter or used as a dairy milk alternative.

4. Pecans: Pecans have a sweet and buttery flavour and are commonly used in desserts like pecan pie. They can also be enjoyed on their own or added to salads and other dishes.

5. Brazil nuts: Brazil nuts have a rich, creamy taste and are known for their high selenium content. They are often eaten raw or used in baking.

6. Pistachios: Pistachios have a slightly sweet and nutty flavour and are often eaten roasted and salted. They are also used in various desserts and confections. In my case their reactions appear immediately with life threatening symptoms but I cut them off completely and you can as well, their reactions to me was constant sneeze and shortage of breath.

7. Hazelnuts: Hazelnuts have a sweet and nutty flavour and are often used in desserts like Nutella or as a flavouring in coffee. They can be eaten raw, roasted, or ground into a paste.

8. Macadamia nuts: Macadamia nuts have a rich, buttery flavour and are often enjoyed roasted or used in baking. They are commonly used in desserts and can also be made into macadamia nut butter.

9. Peanuts: Peanuts are technically legumes, but they are often referred to as nuts. They have a mild, nutty flavour and are commonly eaten roasted or used to make peanut butter.

While those nuts can be tasty and nutritious, there are the large amounts of living things who cannot enjoy them or suffer the consequences of allergic reactions, notice how I said living things and not human beings because all animals who eat in order to survive can have or develop allergies at any given moment and you need to watch out either for yourself or your animals around you

Me myself is allergic to most of them to the point where I shut all of them(nuts)from my list but the most villain is pistachios for me and I get reactions immediately from them, while some of them have to be put on two days window

Two days window goes like this: you eat one nut at a time and then wait for two days watching for red flags, get them on common signs and symptoms

Chapter 3: Signs and Symptoms of Allergies

In this chapter, we will delve into the signs and symptoms of allergies, providing a comprehensive understanding of how allergic reactions manifest in the body. Recognizing these symptoms is vital for timely diagnosis and effective management of allergies.

1. Respiratory Symptoms:

Respiratory symptoms are common in many types of allergies, particularly those related to airborne allergens. These symptoms include:

- Sneezing: Allergies can trigger repeated bouts of sneezing, often accompanied by a runny or congested nose.

- Nasal congestion: Allergic rhinitis, commonly known as hay fever, can cause nasal congestion, making it difficult to breathe through the nose.

- Itchy or watery eyes: Allergies can lead to itchiness and excessive tearing of the eyes, known as allergic conjunctivitis.

- Coughing and wheezing: Allergies can irritate the airways, leading to coughing and wheezing, particularly in individuals with asthma.

2. Skin Reactions:

Allergic reactions can manifest on the skin, resulting in various symptoms:

- Itchy skin: Allergies can cause intense itching, leading to scratching and potential skin damage.

- Hives: Raised, itchy welts on the skin, known as hives or urticaria, can occur as a result of an allergic reaction.

- Eczema: Allergies can worsen or trigger eczema, a chronic skin condition characterised by dry, itchy, and inflamed skin.

3. Gastrointestinal Symptoms:

Some individuals may experience gastrointestinal symptoms as a result of certain food allergies. These symptoms include:

- Nausea and vomiting: Ingesting allergenic foods can lead to feelings of nausea and vomiting.

- Abdominal pain and cramping: Some individuals may experience abdominal discomfort or cramping after consuming specific allergenic foods.

- Diarrhoea: Allergies to certain foods can cause diarrhoea and digestive disturbances.

4. Anaphylaxis:

Anaphylaxis is a severe and potentially life-threatening allergic reaction that can occur within minutes or even seconds after exposure to an allergen. Symptoms of anaphylaxis may include:

- Difficulty breathing: Anaphylaxis can cause airway constriction, making it challenging to breathe.

- Swelling of the face, lips, tongue, or throat: Rapid swelling of these areas can occur during a severe allergic reaction.

- Rapid heartbeat: Anaphylaxis can lead to a sudden increase in heart rate.

- Dizziness or light-headedness: A drop in blood pressure may cause feelings of dizziness or light-headedness.

5. Pimples and blisters:

The foods we eat most of the time impact our health in big way and it shouldn't be ignored because we're what we eat if you hear that quote before and it's true because whatever we eat can manifest itself as a nice skin or problematic skins, so the first things that you will notice when you eat something that's not comfortable with you is a reaction to your skins either as a pimple or blisters and they could be anywhere in your body and when you see it don't ignore the sign, rewind quickly to the last things you consume, it could be liquid or solid form and when you identify it try to write it down and don't eat it for two week and try the other food that you love and cycle goes on until your identify them all.

3.1 Cooking styles matters:

If you cook some foods in a wrong way they will have different reaction on the body and that is what this topic talk about mostly for example if you boils the eggs the egg white will sometimes not be breakdown by your digestive system (bacteria) for some people like me and you might be in this category, I still don't know why but it might have something to do with DNA structure which will be identify in the future endeavour by researchers but now we will focus on how to minimise the reactions by frying the eggs because I know eggs are delicious food

3.2 Diary milk:

It doesn't matter if you cook the milk if your digestive system couldn't breakdown the lactose in milk it will not go well with you therefore you need to eliminate them at all costs and stick with something that is good with your system

You might ask: how do I survive on breastmilk if the milk is problematic for me now? And answer is simple, the milk you are dealing with now are not your mother breastmilk, they are other creature's milks, I'm not trying to villainise milk but if you follow my guide and you identify them as not comfortable with your system, then you are better off without them. Most of the food sometime react differently after they are cooked or before they are cooked which also you need to put in some effort to cook some food in different ways to see what match the best with your bacteria and that is how civilization start with everything we have today and because human are complex compare to other animals that stick with one diets, that is why you need to be your first doctor before the other parties are involved, and don't get me wrong here, you can still go to doctors to seek advice or even treatments but it has to start with you because you are the one who feel the pain and know exactly what start the pain, and you can help yourself quickly than doctors who will wonder around trying to figure out what is the problem while the problem might be what you are eating or drinking

3.3 Others:

Other culprits that you need to look out for are ingredients in which liquor are made of like, sulphites in wine and other ingredients that are not listed here but you can still read the ingredients and find out the triggers, remember that everybody is different including race, gene, and environment they use to live in for example, someone born in Africa and grow up there might have developed the system specific to that environment and if they come to the west, they might experience the changes and sometimes might find it difficult to adapt to the environment therefore I recommend that you pay much attention to what you eat for most part.

It is important to note that the severity and combination of symptoms can vary among individuals, and not everyone may experience all of these symptoms. If you suspect you have allergies or experience any of these symptoms, it is recommended to consult with a healthcare professional for proper diagnosis and guidance.

In the coming chapter, we will explore the various diagnostic methods used to identify allergies, helping individuals gain a clearer understanding of how healthcare professionals determine specific allergenic triggers. Stay tuned for an in-depth exploration of allergy diagnosis techniques and their importance in effective allergy management.

Chapter 4: Diagnosing Allergies:

In this chapter, we will explore the various diagnostic methods used to identify allergies, helping individuals gain a clearer understanding of how healthcare professionals determine specific allergenic triggers. Accurate diagnosis is crucial for effective allergy management and providing appropriate treatment.

1. Medical History:

The first step in diagnosing allergies is obtaining a detailed medical history. Healthcare professionals will ask about your symptoms, their duration, and any potential triggers. They will also inquire about your personal and family history of allergies, as allergies can have a genetic component.

2. Physical Examination:

you can follow the two to five days experimental methods and see which foods is causing a problem and eliminate them, concerning foods and drink or you can go to doctor to identify the non-foods related triggers by physical examination.

During a physical examination, healthcare professionals may assess your overall health and check for specific signs related to allergies, such as swollen nasal passages, red or watery eyes, or skin reactions. The physical examination helps in narrowing down the potential causes of your symptoms.

In Chapter 5, we will explore in detail the different allergy testing methods, their benefits, limitations, and how they aid in diagnosing specific allergens. Stay tuned for an informative exploration of allergy testing techniques and their significance in guiding appropriate

treatments

Chapter 5: Allergy Testing Methods and Their Significance:

In this chapter, we will delve into the different allergy testing methods and their significance in accurately diagnosing specific allergens. These tests play a crucial role in guiding appropriate treatment options and helping individuals effectively manage their allergies.

1. Skin Prick Test:

The skin prick test is a commonly used and reliable method for identifying allergic triggers. During this test, small amounts of suspected allergens are applied to the skin, usually on the forearm or back, using a tiny needle or lancet. If you are allergic to a particular allergen, you will develop a localised allergic reaction at the test site, such as redness, swelling, or itching. The size of the reaction helps determine the severity of the allergy. Skin prick tests are commonly used for airborne allergens like pollen, dust mites, and pet dander, as well as certain food allergens.

2. Specific Ige Blood Test:

The specific Ige blood test measures the levels of specific antibodies called immunoglobulin E (Ige) in your blood. These antibodies are produced in response to allergens. A sample of your blood is sent to a laboratory for analysis, where it is tested for the presence of specific Ige antibodies related to common allergens. The results indicate the likelihood of being allergic to certain substances. The specific Ige blood test is particularly useful when a skin prick test may not be feasible or when multiple allergens need to be tested simultaneously.

3. Elimination Diet:

An elimination diet involves removing suspected allergenic foods from your diet for a period of time, typically a few weeks, and then gradually reintroducing them while monitoring for any allergic reactions. This method helps identify specific food triggers and is especially useful for diagnosing food allergies. It is important to conduct an elimination diet under the guidance of a healthcare professional or a registered dietitian to ensure proper nutrition and avoid unintended nutrient deficiencies.

4. Challenge Tests:

Challenge tests involve controlled exposure to potential allergens under medical supervision. These tests are commonly used when there is uncertainty about a specific allergen or to confirm a diagnosis. Challenge tests can be conducted in various ways, such as inhaling allergens, ingesting food allergens, or applying substances to the skin. The test is closely monitored for any allergic reactions, and the results aid in diagnosing specific allergens.

5. Patch Test:

Patch tests are primarily used to diagnose contact dermatitis, a type of skin allergy caused by direct contact with certain substances. During a patch test, small amounts of suspected allergens are applied to patches that are then placed on your skin, usually on your back. The patches are worn for a specific period, typically 48 hours, and then evaluated for any skin reactions. Patch tests help identify specific substances that may be causing allergic reactions on the skin, such as certain metals, fragrances, or preservatives.

It is important to note that while these allergy testing methods are valuable tools in diagnosing allergies, they may have limitations and should always be interpreted by trained healthcare professionals. Additionally, a comprehensive evaluation of medical history, physical examination, and sometimes additional tests may be necessary to establish an accurate diagnosis.

In Chapter 6, we will explore the various treatment options available for managing allergies, providing insights into both non-pharmacological and pharmacological approaches. Stay tuned for an informative exploration of allergy management strategies and their role in relieving symptoms and preventing allergic reactions options.

Chapter 6: Managing Allergies: Treatment Options:

In this chapter, we will explore the different treatment options available for managing allergies. Effective management is essential in relieving symptoms, preventing allergic reactions, and improving quality of life for individuals with allergies.

1. Allergen Avoidance:

One of the primary strategies for managing allergies is allergen avoidance. This involves identifying and avoiding specific allergens that trigger your allergic reactions. For example, if you have a pollen allergy, you can minimise exposure by staying indoors during peak pollen seasons, using air purifiers, and keeping windows closed. For food allergies, reading labels carefully and avoiding the allergenic food is crucial. Allergen avoidance is an important step in reducing the frequency and severity of allergic symptoms.

2. Medications: I included this in the worst case scenario and I want you to practise the techniques after you get well from the reactions.

Medications are commonly used to alleviate allergy symptoms and manage allergic reactions. Some of the common types of allergy medications include:

a. Antihistamines: Antihistamines work by blocking the effects of histamine, a substance released during allergic reactions. They can help relieve symptoms such as sneezing, itching, and runny nose. Antihistamines are available in both over-the-counter and prescription forms.

b. Nasal corticosteroids: Nasal corticosteroids are effective in reducing inflammation and relieving nasal congestion, sneezing, and itching. They are available as nasal sprays and require a prescription from a healthcare professional.

c. Decongestants: Decongestants help relieve nasal congestion by narrowing blood vessels in the nasal passages. They can be taken orally or used as nasal sprays. It is important to use decongestant nasal sprays for a short duration to avoid rebound congestion.

d. Eye drops: Eye drops containing antihistamines or mast cell stabilisers can provide relief from itchy, watery eyes associated with allergic conjunctivitis.

e. Epinephrine auto-injectors: For individuals with severe allergies and a history of anaphylaxis, an epinephrine auto-injector is a life-saving device. It delivers a dose of epinephrine to quickly reverse severe allergic reactions. It is crucial to carry and know how to use it if prescribed by a healthcare professional.

3. Immunotherapy:

Immunotherapy, also known as allergy shots or allergen immunotherapy, is a long-term treatment option that aims to desensitise the immune system to specific allergens. It involves receiving regular injections containing small amounts of the allergen over a period of time. The treatment gradually helps the immune system become less reactive to the allergen, reducing the severity of allergic symptoms. Immunotherapy is typically recommended for individuals with severe allergies or when allergen avoidance and medication management alone are not sufficient.

4. Sublingual Immunotherapy (SLIT):

Sublingual immunotherapy (SLIT) is an alternative to allergy shots. It involves placing allergen extracts under the tongue and allowing them to be absorbed. This method can be self-administered at home after an initial evaluation and prescription from a healthcare professional. SLIT is available for certain allergens, such as grass pollen, dust mites, and ragweed. It can be a convenient option for individuals who are unable to undergo allergy shots.

5. Education and Support:

Education and support play a vital role in managing allergies. Understanding your allergies, knowing how to read labels, recognizing potential triggers, and learning proper medication use are essential. Allergy support groups and resources can provide valuable information, tips, and a sense of community for individuals managing allergies. Healthcare professionals, such as allergists or immunologists, can provide guidance, education, and support tailored to your specific needs.

In the next chapter, we will explore practical tips and lifestyle modifications that can complement allergy management strategies and help individuals reduce their exposure to allergens. Stay tuned for valuable insights on creating an allergy-friendly environment and implementing healthy habits to minimise allergic reactions.

Chapter 7: Creating an Allergy-Friendly Environment:

In this chapter, we will explore practical tips and lifestyle modifications that can help individuals create an allergy-friendly environment. By implementing these strategies, you can reduce your exposure to allergens and minimise the risk of allergic reactions.

1. Keep Your Living Space Clean:

Regular cleaning is essential in maintaining an allergy-friendly environment. Dust, pet dander, and other allergens can accumulate on surfaces, carpets, and furniture. Vacuuming with a HEPA filter, dusting with a damp cloth, and washing bedding regularly can help reduce allergen levels.

2. Control Indoor Humidity:

Maintaining optimal indoor humidity levels can prevent the growth of mould and dust mites, which are common allergenic triggers. Use a dehumidifier in damp areas, such as basements, and ensure proper ventilation in bathrooms and kitchens to minimise moisture accumulation.

3. Minimise Exposure to Dust Mites:

Dust mites are microscopic organisms that thrive in warm and humid environments. To reduce exposure:

a. Encase mattresses, pillows, and bedding in allergen-proof covers.

b. Wash bedding in hot water regularly.

c. Avoid using thick curtains and opt for blinds or washable curtains instead.

d. Remove stuffed animals or wash them frequently in hot water.

4. Control Pet Allergens:

If you have allergies to pet dander, consider the following:

a. Keep pets out of your bedroom and other areas where you spend a significant amount of time.

b. Regularly bathe and groom your pets to reduce dander levels.

c. Vacuum and dust frequently to minimise pet dander accumulation.

5. Manage Pollen Exposure:

Pollen allergies can be challenging, especially during peak seasons. To minimise exposure:

a. Monitor local pollen forecasts and try to stay indoors during high pollen counts.

b. Keep windows closed and use air purifiers with HEPA filters to reduce pollen indoors.

c. Shower and change clothes after spending time outdoors to remove any pollen residue.

6. Create a Healthy Bedroom:

Your bedroom should be a sanctuary free from allergens. Consider the following:

a. Use hypoallergenic pillows and bedding.

b. Avoid plush carpets and opt for hardwood or laminate flooring.

c. Keep the bedroom clean and well-ventilated.

d. Consider using an air purifier with a HEPA filter to improve air quality.

7. Implement Healthy Habits:

In addition to managing your environment, adopting healthy habits can support allergy management:

a. Maintain good hand hygiene to prevent the spread of allergens from surfaces to your face.

b. Avoid smoking and exposure to second-hand smoke, as it can worsen allergy symptoms.

c. Eat a balanced diet rich in fruits, vegetables, and omega-3 fatty acids, which can help support a healthy immune system.

d. Stay hydrated to keep nasal passages moist and alleviate congestion.

By implementing these tips and lifestyle modifications, you can create an allergy-friendly environment that supports your allergy management efforts. Remember that allergies are unique to each individual, so it is important to identify your specific triggers and tailor your environment accordingly. Don't break your wallets, just start with what you have and practice the identify and eliminate methods.

In the final chapter, we will discuss strategies for preventing allergies and reducing the risk of developing new allergies. Stay tuned for valuable insights on allergy prevention and maintaining long-term allergy management.

Bonus: have fun

Mental telepathy:

People of all ages have argued about this phenomenon whether the mental telepathy exists or not, I don't have a conclusive evidence but I have the experiment which I experience myself and as you might guess, the human species has one consciousness that contains five senses and the other senses that is shrouded in mystery call six senses or third man syndrome and just because you can't prove something doesn't mean it doesn't exist.

I myself as a student of universe, I experience a lot of many things that are not explanatory but could be experienced and no evidence, I accept that the mental telepathy is real but just not advanced like telephone and other sources of communication

Here is the analogy of how I think it works:

You, the initiator of communication begins with thoughts of other person, whether it be oh I miss that guy or when can I see him/her again and then the other person that you are thinking about is alerted by optical fibre (God mode)that you are trying to get in contact with them and they didn't pick, so if the other person likes you or use to think about you then they are likely to get your contact through mental telepathy fibre and they will begin to think about you leading to any of you getting to make the actual contact and if other person doesn't have the same feelings then the chances are slim for them to get your message. end you can add your experience or comment if you have the same experience

The problem itself:

Whenever anything occurred whether it be headache, acne, tiredness, and anything that affect the body in an annoying way, what you can do is not rush and take medicine instead what you suppose to do is to ask yourself what was the last food you eat or any last thing you put in your mouth whether it be food, medicine, any type of drinks, and other ingestible things you took in that passage of time please conduct thoroughly before you proceed with any help from third party unless it's emergency

The food cycle:

When you eat the food the researchers show that it takes 8 hours for food to go to your system and 36 hours to go through elimination cycle and according to my research when it comes to any allergies that may appear in your system it take immediate effect or 1 hour for reaction to occur, whether it be dairy product reaction or any type of nuts reaction and bear in mind that different people have different experience with any type of food, the goal here is to determine which food is your system doesn't like and eliminate that and don't worry there are variety of food to eat and live your normal life, just know that anything that you put in your mouth and upset your system is not good for you no matter how good it is, whether it be alcohol or any type of food and that is the universal facts, now the choice is yours whether to continue ingesting the dread or stop it and embrace your new life

Top 11:

 Foods That Can Cause Acne & What To Eat For Clear Skin and you still need to watch that food closely at all time.

Simple changes in your dietary habits can give you clear, glowing, and healthy skin.

The relationship between food and acne is controversial. There are contradicting studies in this regard, with some even claiming to have zeroed in on foods that cause acne. However, we know that our nutrient intake impacts our skin health, and our diet plays a major role in maintaining our skin.

A study conducted in France tried to determine whether diet has any impact on the prevalence of acne in adults. Out of 24,452 participants, 11 324 (46%) reported past or current acne, 3576 (32%) believed diet was a factor, 3503 (31%) believed diet was not a factor, and 4195 (37%) were unsure of whether diet was a factor. It showed that acne can occur 1.43 and 3.90 times more due to carbohydrate and saturated fat intake respectively.

While food alone cannot cause acne, certain foods can worsen your existing acne – and more research is required to establish the connection starting from boil eggs to eleven food that you will read through here.

List Of Top Foods That Cause Acne

1. Refined Grains And Sugar

A study involving 64 participants with moderate to severe acne found that those with acne consumed a greater amount of carbohydrates. Moreover, these participants with acne also had high amounts of insulin-like growth factor-1 (a hormone that causes high sebum production, which usually peaks during puberty).

Another study found that frequent intake of sugar could lead to acne development in adolescents

Rice noodles, pasta, and noodles made of white flour

Bread, cereals, cakes, pastries, and cookies made of white flour

Sugary beverages

Sweeteners such as honey, maple syrup, cane sugar

2. Dairy Products

A study reviewing the high school diet of 47,355 women found a positive connection between acne and intake of whole and skimmed milk. Other dairy products, such as cream cheese and cottage cheese, were also found to worsen acne.

Another case-control study evaluated 44 individuals with acne vulgaris and 44 controls for three months. They found that individuals with acne more often ate food with a high glycaemic index load compared to the controls. They drank milk and had ice cream more frequently than the controls.

A beauty blogger who had a history of severe acne spoke about how milk had been a major culprit. She said, "Cutting cow milk out a few years ago cleared up 90% of my body acne and I always attributed this to the positive effects of reducing my hormone consumption."

3. Fast Food Or Junk Food

A study evaluating the prevalence of acne in adolescents found that those with acne lacked healthy dietary habits. The researchers concluded that frequent intake of fast foods like fatty foods, burgers, sausages, cakes, pastries, and sugar might increase the risk of acne or aggravate it.

4. Foods With High Levels of Omega-6 Fats

A typical western diet contains high levels of omega-6 fatty acids and lower levels of omega-3s. Omega-6 fatty acids are found in most of the vegetable and cooking oils, and most processed foods are cooked in these oils.

You don't have to eliminate the intake of omega-6 fats. You can control your consumption of processed foods and foods made in vegetable oils. Choose oils that are low in omega-6 fatty acids. These include olive oil, coconut oil, and palm oil. Avoid intake of oils high in omega-6 fatty acids, including sunflower, soybean, and cottonseed oils.

5. Whey Protein Powder

Whey protein is the liquid left behind after the milk is curdled and separated during the cheese-making process. Although whey is rich in amino acids, whey protein has been linked to increased acne in gym-going adolescents who take it. Though the acne (especially on the trunk) could be caused only by perspiration, more research is warranted to establish the causes.

Milk and milk products can increase IGF-1 receptors and the production of hormones like progesterone and oestrogen. It is believed that they may contribute to acne, though more research is warranted to understand the mechanism behind it.

6. Non-Organic Meat

Natural or synthetic steroid hormone drugs (including progesterone, oestrogen, and testosterone) are often used to increase the growth rate of animals. This is done to get them ready faster for human consumption and has been approved by the FDA.

Consuming such meats may also trigger acne by increasing the action of androgens and Insulin-like Growth Factor.

7. Caffeine And Alcohol

A study states that coffee reduces insulin sensitivity. This means your blood sugar levels stay high for a longer period than usual after you drink coffee. This may increase inflammation and worsen your acne.

Another study evaluated the diet of Kitava people who did not have acne. Their diet involved the minimal intake of coffee, alcohol, sugar, oils, and dairy products.

8. Canned Food

Frozen, canned, and pre-cooked meals can be considered processed foods. These often contain added ingredients, such as sweeteners, oils, spices, and preservatives, which are used as flavourings. Ready-to-eat foods and excessively sugary or spicy foods are usually heavily processed and can contribute to acne.

9. Fried Food

Potato chips, fries, burgers, and other processed and fried foods can also cause acne. These also include other high-glycaemic foods that raise your blood sugar levels quickly, causing inflammatory conditions like acne

10. Energy Drinks

Energy drinks contain high levels of sugar and can increase blood glucose levels. In one study, intake of sugar from soft drinks was found to increase acne risk Any sugary drink can increase your risk of acne. Hence, So avoid drinking excessive amounts of sugary energy drinks and soft drinks.

11. Chocolate

Research indicates that the intake of chocolate is associated with an increase in the severity of acne in people with acne-prone skin. A study conducted by Chulalongkorn University, Thailand found that the consumption of 25 grams of 99% dark chocolate for 4 weeks increased the number of acne lesions in acne-prone male subjects. Another study published in the Journal of Clinical and Aesthetic Dermatology observed that the consumption of dark chocolate can increase the risk of acne development by promoting bacterial colonisation on the surface of facial skin. However, it is unclear if these effects alone are sufficient to trigger acne development and more research is warranted in this regard and also different foods react differently to different people, some of these foods might not be bad for your system, that is why you need to follow the techniques that I give you.

Chapter 8: Where do allergies most likely show up?

Allergic reactions can manifest in various parts of the body, depending on the allergen involved and individual factors. Some common areas where allergic reactions may appear include:

1. **Skin**: Skin reactions are quite common in allergic responses and can include hives (raised, red, itchy welts), eczema (dry, itchy, inflamed skin e.g. pimple, blackheads and blisters), and general itching or rash.
2. **Respiratory System**: Allergens like pollen, dust mites, pet dander, and certain foods can trigger allergic reactions in the respiratory system, leading to symptoms such as sneezing, runny or stuffy nose, coughing, wheezing, and difficulty breathing.

3. **Eyes**: Allergic reactions can cause redness, itching, watering, and swelling of the eyes, known as allergic conjunctivitis.
4. **Digestive System**: Ingested allergens, such as certain foods or medications, can lead to symptoms such as nausea, vomiting, abdominal pain, diarrhoea, or even anaphylaxis.
5. **Mouth and Throat**: Some allergic reactions can cause itching or swelling in the mouth, lips, tongue, or throat, which can lead to difficulty swallowing or breathing.
6. **Whole Body**: In severe cases, allergic reactions can cause a systemic response known as anaphylaxis, which can lead to a drop in blood pressure, loss of consciousness, and even death if not treated promptly.

The specific symptoms and affected areas can vary widely among individuals and depend on factors such as the type and severity of the allergy, the route of exposure to the allergen, and individual sensitivity

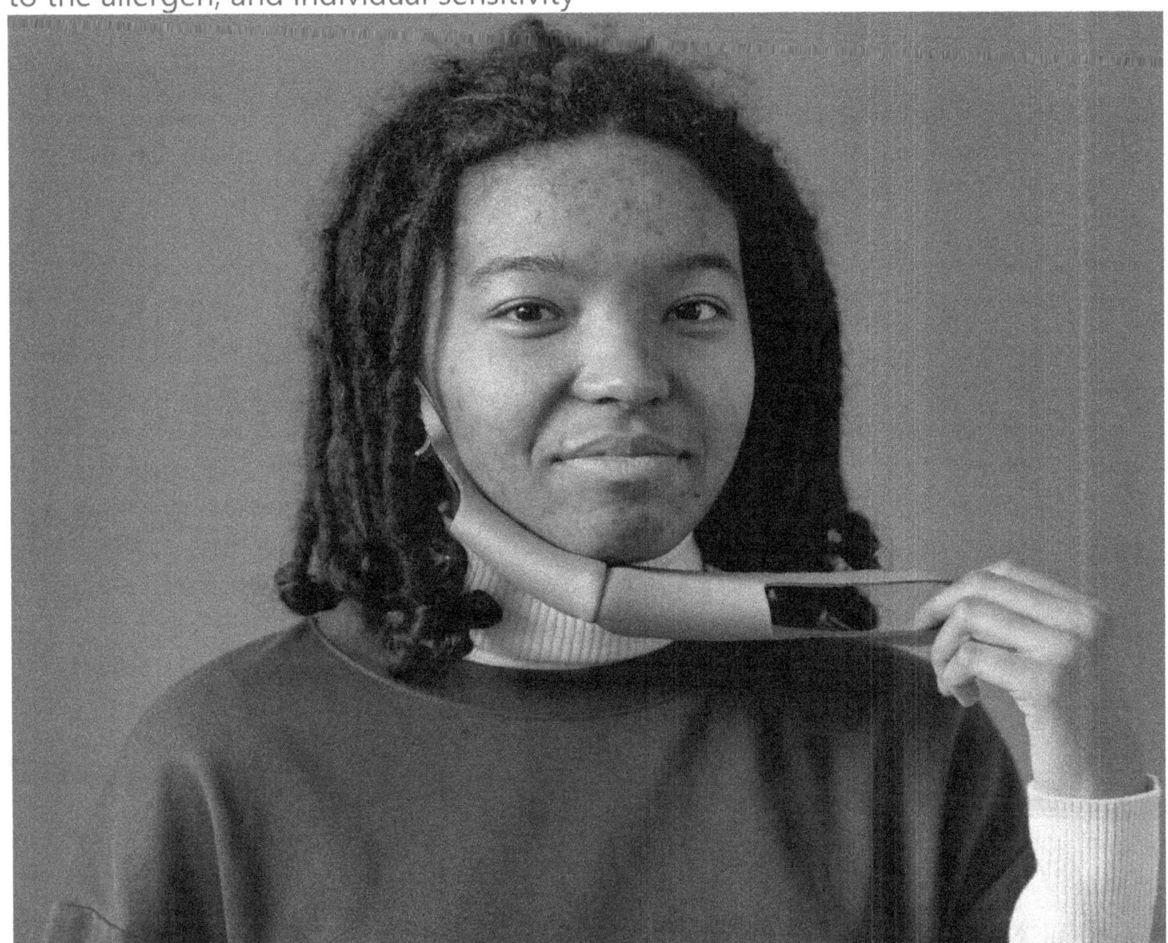

This young girl is on her post allergic state and she's on healing process which you can see now

While none of the studies are conclusive, and there is a need for more research, avoiding certain foods is more likely to help reduce the risk of acne. At the same time, adding certain other foods to your diet can help make your skin clear and healthy.

What To Eat To Keep Your Skin Clear

Here are a few foods that you can add to your diet to keep your skin clear and potentially prevent acne:

1. Foods Rich In Omega-3 Fatty Acids

Unlike omega-6 fatty acids, omega-3 fatty acids have anti-inflammatory properties. Those on a diet high in omega-3 fatty acids were found to have lower levels of acne. Hence, eat more foods like salmon, sardines, herring, canola oil, and other fish, like tuna, catfish, shrimps, and clams. These help increase your intake of the omega-3 fats.

2. Probiotics

Probiotics produce antibacterial proteins and inhibit the growth of P. acnes and Sauers bacteria . Both these bacteria are known to cause acne.

3. Green Tea

Green tea contains polyphenols that act as anti-inflammatory and antimicrobial agents. Some evidence shows that these polyphenols help reduce excess sebum production and inhibit the growth

.

4. Turmeric

Turmeric contains curcumin, a compound responsible for its therapeutic benefits. Whether you take it orally or apply it topically, turmeric can help in the treatment of skin conditions like acne .

5. Foods Rich In Vitamins A, D, E, And Zinc

These vitamins help maintain skin health. A deficiency of these essential vitamins could often lead to acne. You can consume fried eggs, not boil eggs, broccoli, fatty fish like mackerel and tuna, nuts and seeds, and legumes.

6. The Mediterranean Diet

The Mediterranean diet involves a high intake of proteins, fresh vegetables, whole grains, herbs, spices, seafood, seeds, legumes, and extra virgin olive oil. Foods like cheese, poultry, and eggs are eaten in moderation, while processed foods, refined grains, and sugary beverages are to be excluded completely. Following the Mediterranean diet was found to reduce the risk of acne. If you are allergic to gluten you may have millet as a healthy whole-grain option.

Diet plays a crucial role in maintaining overall skin health. A holistic approach is necessary to reduce acne and boost skin health. Yes, it can be difficult to make dietary changes, but you can always start slow. Try cutting down on junk food and follow a balanced lifestyle to achieve clearer skin.

Bonus:

Baldness is caused by wearing cap and headgear that has hardcore in the forehead, it heat it up and causes resistance making hair recede and falls out eventually resulting in baldness and sometimes you need to make more observations to find out more but this one is the culprit of all time,

Some causes include:

Hormones

Age

Bad barbers

D/R/U/G/S

Stress

Alopecia areata

Autoimmune disease

Genetics

Hypothyroidism

Hair care

Infection

Medical conditions

Nutritional deficiencies

Stress or shock

Androgenetic alopecia

Hair damage

Injury

Obesity

Scalp infection

Instead wear a soft headgear so short and precise

Chapter 9: fasting for cell recycling.

1. Metabolic Health

- **Improved Insulin Sensitivity**: Fasting can help enhance insulin sensitivity, which may reduce the risk of type 2 diabetes.
- **Weight Loss**: Fasting can lead to calorie reduction, promoting weight loss and reducing body fat.

2. Cellular and Molecular Benefits

- **Autophagy**: Fasting induces autophagy, a process where the body cleans out damaged cells and regenerates new ones, potentially reducing the risk of various diseases.
- **Hormone Regulation**: Fasting influences the production of certain hormones, like increasing norepinephrine, which helps mobilize fat for energy.

3. Cardiovascular Health

- **Reduced Inflammation**: Fasting can lower inflammation levels, which is beneficial for heart health.
- **Improved Cholesterol Levels**: Fasting can lead to reductions in bad cholesterol (LDL) and triglycerides.

4. Brain Health

- **Enhanced Cognitive Function**: Fasting can improve brain function and reduce the risk of neurodegenerative diseases like Alzheimer's and Parkinson's.
- **Increased Neurogenesis**: Fasting may stimulate the production of new neurons and protect the brain from damage.

5. Longevity

- **Life Extension**: Studies in animals suggest that fasting can extend lifespan and delay the onset of age-related diseases.

6. Mental and Emotional Well-being

- **Improved Mood and Mental Clarity**: Many people report better mood, increased alertness, and mental clarity during fasting periods.
- **Stress Resistance**: Fasting may improve the body's ability to handle stress by enhancing resilience at the cellular level.

7. Digestive Health

- **Gut Health**: Fasting gives the digestive system a break, which can improve gut health and reduce symptoms of bloating and discomfort.

Types of Fasting

- **Intermittent Fasting (IF)**: Alternating periods of eating and fasting, such as the 16/8 method (16 hours fasting, 8 hours eating).
- **Time-Restricted Eating**: Eating all meals within a specific window each day, such as 10 hours.
- **Extended Fasting**: Fasting for more than 24 hours, such as 48 or 72 hours.

Safety and Considerations

- **Medical Supervision**: It's important to consult with a healthcare provider before starting a fasting regimen, especially for individuals with underlying health conditions.
- **Hydration**: Drinking water is crucial during fasting to prevent dehydration.
- **Nutrient Intake**: Ensuring adequate nutrient intake during eating periods to avoid deficiencies.

  Fasting is for everyone and more importantly for your health

  It's a little bit uncomfortable but it is worth it for your longevity and healthy life, some symptoms are lack of energy, headache, and bit of discomfort but you can make your surrounding aware of this actions so that they can not be confused if you slipped out of your characters, hopefully not.

  And if you were bias thinking that it is for religious people only, then you get that idea wrong I know this because I was bias myself but the more I research the more I debunk many myths and misconceptions

Chapter 10: Training to refer the damaged tissues

Training stimulates the body through a variety of physiological processes that help it adapt to the demands placed upon it during exercise. Here are some key ways in which training stimulates the body:

1. **Muscle Contraction and Strength**: Training, particularly resistance training, stimulates muscle Fibers to contract against resistance. This leads to microscopic damage to muscle Fibers, which the body repairs and rebuilds, resulting in muscle growth and increased strength over time.
2. **Cardiovascular System**: Cardiovascular training, such as running, cycling, or swimming, stimulates the heart and lungs to work harder to supply oxygen to the muscles. This improves cardiovascular fitness by increasing the heart's efficiency, improving circulation, and enhancing lung capacity.
3. **Metabolism**: Training can increase metabolism, both during and after exercise. Intense exercise can boost metabolic rate temporarily,
4. and over time, regular exercise can lead to increased muscle mass, which further elevates basal metabolic rate.
5. **Bone Density**: Weight-bearing exercises such as walking, jogging, and strength training stimulate bone remodelling, leading to increased bone density and strength. This helps prevent bone loss and reduces the risk of osteoporosis.

6. **Neurological Adaptations**: Training can lead to neurological adaptations that improve motor coordination, balance, and proprioception. These adaptations result from the brain's ability to fine-tune movement patterns in response to repeated practice and feedback.

7. **Hormonal Response**: Exercise stimulates the release of various hormones, including endorphins (which reduce pain perception and induce feelings of well-being), adrenaline (which increases heart rate and blood pressure during intense exercise), and growth hormone (which stimulates tissue growth and repair).

8. **Mental Health**: Regular exercise has been shown to have numerous mental health benefits, including reducing stress, anxiety, and depression. Exercise stimulates the release of neurotransmitters like serotonin and dopamine, which contribute to improved mood and overall well-being.

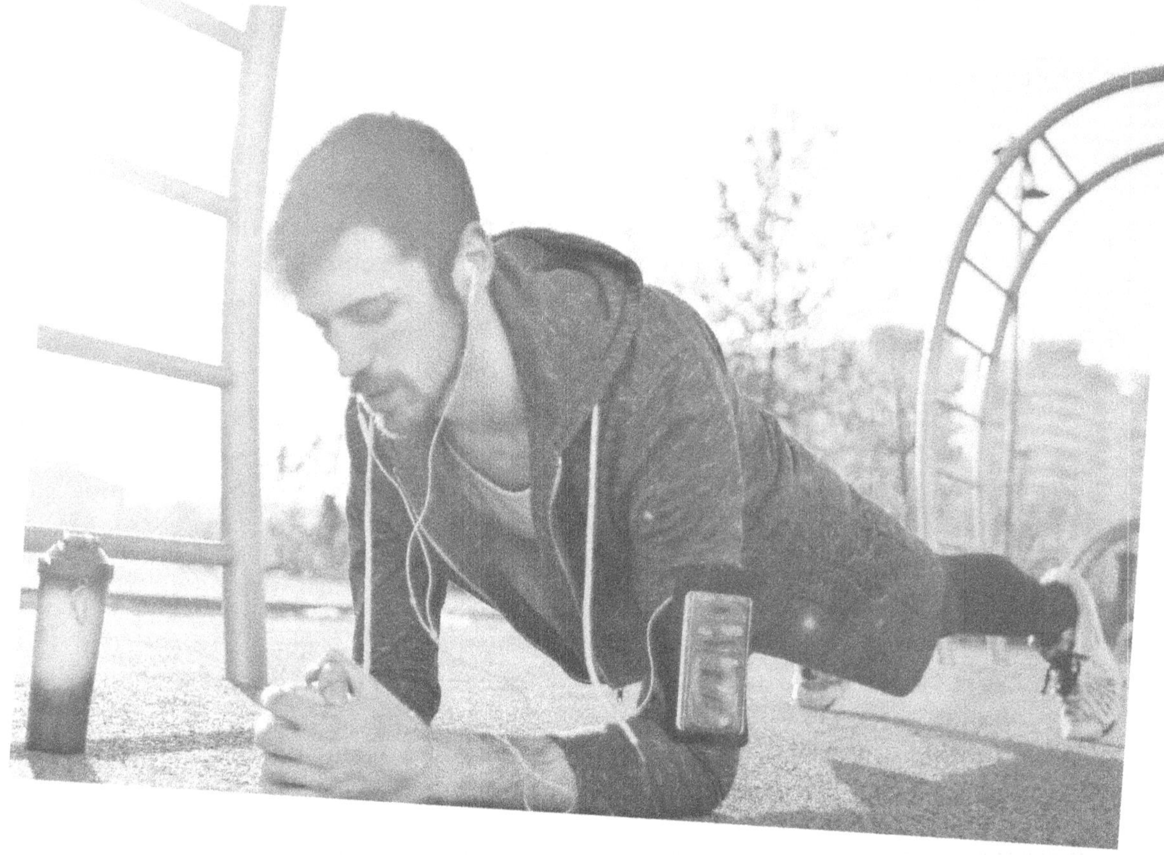

Overall, training stimulates the body by challenging its various systems and prompting adaptive responses that lead to improved physical fitness, health, and performance.

Chapter 11: drinking water (staying hydrated)

Staying hydrated is crucial for maintaining overall health and well-being. Here are the key reasons why proper hydration is important:

1. Supports Physical Performance

- **Endurance and Strength**: Adequate hydration helps maintain strength, power, and endurance during exercise and physical activities.
- **Temperature Regulation**: Water helps regulate body temperature through sweating, preventing overheating during workouts.

2. Cognitive Function and Mood

- **Mental Clarity**: Dehydration can impair cognitive functions such as concentration, alertness, and short-term memory.
- **Mood Stability**: Proper hydration helps maintain a balanced mood, reducing feelings of irritability and anxiety.

3. Digestive Health

- **Aids Digestion**: Water is essential for the digestive process, helping dissolve nutrients and facilitate their absorption.
- **Prevents Constipation**: Adequate water intake helps prevent constipation by softening stools and promoting regular bowel movements.

4. Kidney Function and Detoxification

- **Waste Removal**: Kidneys need water to filter waste products from the blood and excrete them through urine.
- **Prevents Kidney Stones**: Proper hydration reduces the risk of developing kidney stones by diluting minerals and salts in urine.

5. Joint and Muscle Health

- **Lubricates Joints**: Water acts as a lubricant for joints, reducing the risk of joint pain and disorders.
- **Muscle Function**: Hydration helps maintain the balance of electrolytes, which are critical for muscle contraction and function.

6. Skin Health

- **Moisturizes Skin**: Adequate hydration helps keep skin moisturized, improving its elasticity and reducing the appearance of wrinkles.
- **Promotes Healing**: Water aids in the healing process of skin injuries and supports overall skin health.

7. Maintains Blood Pressure and Heart Health

- **Circulation**: Water helps maintain adequate blood volume, which is essential for healthy blood pressure and circulation.
- **Heart Efficiency**: Proper hydration supports the heart's ability to pump blood more effectively, reducing cardiovascular strain.

8. Regulates Body Temperature

- **Sweating**: Water is crucial for the body's sweating mechanism, which helps cool the body and maintain a stable internal temperature.

9. Boosts Immune Function

- **Fluid Balance**: Hydration supports the optimal function of all bodily systems, including the immune system, enhancing the body's ability to fight off infections.

10. Weight Management

- **Appetite Control**: Drinking water can help control appetite and prevent overeating, as thirst is often mistaken for hunger.
- **Metabolism Boost**: Proper hydration can boost metabolic rate, aiding in weight management efforts.

Practical Tips for Staying Hydrated:

- **Drink Regularly**: Consume water regularly throughout the day, not just when you're thirsty.
- **Eat Hydrating Foods**: Include fruits and vegetables with high water content in your diet.
- **Monitor Urine Colour**: Aim for light yellow urine, which typically indicates proper hydration.
- **Carry a Water Bottle**: Keep a reusable water bottle with you to make it easier to drink water throughout the day.
- **Set Reminders**: Use phone apps or alarms to remind you to drink water at regular intervals. Like me I'm using my phone to remind me whenever I forget because sometimes you could be busy with many tasks, also having a stainless steel with you is the best way to get hydrated easily.

Chapter 12: Protecting the skins.

Protecting your skin from the sun is crucial for preventing sunburn, premature aging, and reducing the risk of skin cancer. Here are several effective strategies to protect your skin from the sun and because there are many misconception about the skins differences that's not true in this case because sun can burn every skins out there and speed up the aging process

1. Use Sunscreen

- **Broad-Spectrum Protection:** Choose a sunscreen that offers broad-spectrum protection against both UVA and UVB rays.
- **SPF 30 or Higher:** Use a sunscreen with an SPF of at least 30.
- **Water-Resistant:** If you are swimming or sweating, choose a water-resistant sunscreen.
- **Reapply Regularly:** Apply sunscreen 15 minutes before going outside and reapply every two hours, or more frequently if swimming or sweating.

2. Wear Protective Clothing

- **Long-Sleeved Shirts and Pants:** opt for clothing that covers more skin.
- **UPF Clothing:** Consider clothing with an Ultraviolet Protection Factor (UPF) rating.
- **Wide-Brimmed Hats:** Wear hats that shade your face, ears, and neck.
- **Sunglasses:** Protect your eyes with sunglasses that block 100% of UVA and UVB rays.

3. Seek Shade

- **Avoid Peak Sun Hours:** Stay indoors or in the shade during peak sun hours, typically between 10 AM and 4 PM.
- **Use Umbrellas and Shade Structures:** Use umbrellas, canopies, or other shade structures when outdoors.

4. Be Mindful of Reflective Surfaces

- **Water, Sand, and Snow:** Be aware that these surfaces can reflect and intensify the sun's rays, increasing the risk of sunburn.

5. Regular Skin Checks

- **Monitor Skin for Changes:** Regularly check your skin for any new moles or changes in existing moles.
- **Consult a Dermatologist:** See a dermatologist annually for a professional skin exam.

6. Hydration and Skincare

- **Stay Hydrated:** Drink plenty of water to keep your skin hydrated.
- **Moisturize:** Use a moisturizer to keep your skin from drying out, especially after sun exposure. And avoid the heavy make-up in your daily routine and increase the exercise.

7. Avoid Tanning Beds

- **Steer Clear of Artificial Tanning:** Tanning beds emit harmful UV radiation that can increase the risk of skin cancer.

8. Dietary Considerations

- **Antioxidants:** Consume foods rich in antioxidants, like fruits and vegetables, which can help protect your skin from sun damage.

Also the reverse is true about foods, if you eat the food that might be harmful to your gut system like mentioned in top 11 food that are prove to expose damage to your skins e.g. sugar is the devil in disguised of sweet and kills slowly, so if you are to take sugar make sure you take it with caution because it's the only innocent but harmful legal drug in the shelves

And also overeating can reduced the digestive system response, causing your skin to stress out and increase the aging process that's why you see poor people aging like fine wines and rich people having many health issues because they can afford to buy more sugar foods and constantly eating due to the availability of everything, but if you are a rich person you can still read this book and stay in control of your health

Cold ❄

cold is something that you will always encounter in almost any situation but the most common problems is the after shower if you didn't dry yourself well enough with towels , you are likely to catch the cold or if you go out immediately after shower, instead relax for a few minutes and make to wear the correct gear like scarp, soft hat, and warm jacket.

Showers and cleaning yourself

Human skin sheds continuously as part of the natural process of cell turnover. The outer layer of the skin, called the epidermis, is composed mainly of dead skin cells that eventually slough off and are replaced by new cells from the lower layers of the epidermis. On average, it's estimated that the outer layer of the skin completely renews itself approximately every 28 to 30 days for adults. However, this process can vary depending on factors such as age, health, and environmental conditions. Therefore you need to clean yourself more often in the right way and the effective to do so is using the luffa, and well trim fingers are the best exfoliator but you need to be gentle with them not to hurt yourself and with practice you get better over time and when drying

Contents

1. **Metabolic Health** 20

2. **Cellular and Molecular Benefits** 20

3. **Cardiovascular Health** 21

4. **Brain Health** 21

5. **Longevity** 21

6. **Mental and Emotional Well-being** 21

7. **Digestive Health** 21

Types of Fasting..21

Safety and Considerations 21

1. Supports Physical Performance 24

2. Cognitive Function and Mood 24

3. Digestive Health 24

4. Kidney Function and Detoxification 24

5. Joint and Muscle Health 24

6. Skin Health..24

7. Maintains Blood Pressure and Heart Health 25

8. Regulates Body Temperature 25

9. Boosts Immune Function 25

10. Weight Management 25

Practical Tips for Staying Hydrated:...25

1. Use Sunscreen 25

2. Wear Protective Clothing..26

3. Seek Shade..26

4. Be Mindful of Reflective Surfaces 26

5. Regular Skin Checks 26

6. Hydration and Skincare 26

7. Avoid Tanning Beds 26

8. Dietary Considerations..26

yourself with towel, don't rub your face instead just wipe with your normal hands after you dry your body, and moisturise your face immediately to lock in the moisture

Conclusion:

I will conclude that by saying thank you my friend for reading the book and I hope you will follow this technique and apply them to your life and I hope your life get better and please I will be happy if you recommend this book to your friends, all the best. Always look inside for answers to your life.

I might not know all the foods around the world because there are variety of foods that people consume in different countries but applying the two days window techniques or 30 days window if you want to confirm it 100% and eliminate it totally. It's the eye opening process and helpful if you can apply it correctly.

your one month calendar here: with all the good food that will stick with you and the food that will go.

Your gratitude for your journey here:

Author details:

Contact us at:

Email: Akoldjuan@gmail.com

ALSO follow us on Amazon through Daniel Akol Kuan account